Needbased Eating

Liv Larsson

friare LIV

Mjösjölidvägen 477, 946 40 Svensbyn
info@friareliv.se
www.friareliv.se

Need based eating by Liv Larsson translated from Friheten på botten av chipspåsen by Liv Larsson

Friare Liv
Mjösjölidvägen 477
946 40 Svensbyn
Sweden
Phone: +46 911- 24 11 44
info@friareliv.se
www.friareliv.se/eng

Author: Liv Larsson
Translation: Liv Larsson
Proofreading: Belinda Poropudas
Layout: Kay Rung
Illustrations: Vilhelm PH Nilsson: vilhelm@uppsalanaturbete.se

ISBN:978-91-87489-34-1 Print edition
ISBN 978-91-87489-35-8 E-pub edition

Content

Foreword

Throughout my life I have tried to find some way to experience a sense of choice in relation-ship to food. During my childhood, I was often frustrated by being told that eating everything on my plate was important, both at school and at home, even when I was stuffed. This period in my life was followed by periods of starvation and periods of binge eating in my teenage years.

After being diagnosed as anorexic and bulimic, I finally managed to create a sane balance between weight, eating and exercise. Yet a lot of the time I still searched for freedom at "the bottom of the chip bag" or in some diet. During more than three decades of my life I was focusing on controlling both my weight and the food I ate. In those years I thought that if I could just learn about different kinds of food, calorie consumption and how to eat "right," all would feel okay.

Countless books and health magazines that focused on this topic passed through my hands. I constantly went through health cures, detoxes or diets. I managed to keep a weight that was quite stable and was never really overweight (although my head said something different most of the time), but no matter how much I learned, the balance I longed for never appeared. I was ob¬sessed by what I should eat, what I should stop eating, and how to become slimmer. At the same time I was longing to feel free and not having my whole life revolving around these issues.[1] Then I discovered Nonviolent Communication (NVC) and I decided to let it shape my lifestyle and my work.[2]

As NVC focuses on human needs, it was natural for me to explore the needs I wanted to meet through eating. I realized how often I put something in my mouth for reasons other than for my needs for energy or nutrition. It made me curious to see if I could find other- more fulfilling - ways to meet these needs. Since then, I have experienced a growing freedom around eating and my choices of food and exercise.

---

1. The term Orthorexia is used to describe an excessive focus on health and control over food and exercise.
2. Read more about NVC - Nonviolent Communication at www.cnvc.org

Needbased Eating
Liv Larsson

Several books - including Sylvia Haskvitz's Eat By choice, Not By Habit and Paul McKenna's I Can Make you Thin - have meant a lot to me in my search for a natural way to relate to food and my body. Now, as I write this book, it is because I have come to a place within myself where I can live up to what I am writing about. Besides, I know that it can also be a support for others, as I discovered when testing much of the content with a group of people I coached for quite a while. People who have benefited greatly from what has now become this little book, so it feels great to now see it come into print.

This is not a book about dieting or about how to lose weight. It is about how to make friends with your body and with your impulses around hunger and satiety. It is about finding a way to live, with which you can feel pleased.

If you find any pointing fingers or suggestions that you must do certain things I suggest in this book - throw it out immediately (or use it as toilet paper). Durable health and balance is not achieved through coercion. The balance you experience when you force yourself disappears as soon as you let go of control. Two things prevented me from completing the writing of this book earlier. One was worrying about being a part in making people - especially women - to have even more thoughts about how important it is to be thin. A tremendous amount of energy is already being used in focusing on appearance. What I want to do is to help people to find freedom, pleasure, and balance in their eating and in their life.

The second obstacle for me in writing this book was a variation of the first. I myself have been focused on becoming or "being thin" for many years. Even as I saw how absurd it is that so many women spend such a tremendous amount of time and energy in worrying over, learning about, and trying out different diets, I have been doing just the same thing. I have often asked myself who would I have been if I had not had this mania about not being thin enough. What could I have put all that time and effort into. Now, when I seldom worry about my weight, I know that it has been replaced by an inner peace that I wish for everyone, women and men alike.

Dilemmas Around Eating

Many of us are not friends with our bodies, which take different expressions for different people. We do not know how to balance health with pleasure, structure with freedom of choice, freedom with faith. A natural behavior like eating has become unnecessarily complicated and tons of books about this "problem" with food have been written.

Many people have lost the ability to balance "energy in" and "energy out" and to find a healthy and easy way to eat. Many yearn to experience freedom around food, body and weight. Do you recognize yourself in these dilemmas?

- You yearn for a sense of autonomy and freedom around the choice of food.

- You want to trust that you are eating in a way that supports your health.

- You often have thoughts of wanting to lose weight but do not act to do so, or jump from one diet to the other.

- You find it challenging to find motivation to change your thoughts and habits around food and weight, even if you are not fully satisfied with your current choices.

- You often eat more than you want and need.

- You sometimes think of your body and weight in a way that feels stressful.

- You have thoughts like: I just cannot stop once I've started, I've got such bad character, I will lose control, I have lost control.

- Breaking an attempt to follow some kind of diet you sometimes have thoughts like: "I've already ruined this attempt to eat healthily, so I might as well just give up."

Your Eating Habits

Needs are central to the ideas in this book. When I use the word need, I mean inner motivational forces that are universally human, something that all people of all ages and cultures have in common. Our needs motivate us to act. Whatever we do, we might see these actions as attempts to meet our needs.

Sometimes our needs are met, sometimes not. Most of us also eat to meet other needs than those of nutrition and energy. Sometimes this leads to undesirable consequences, especially if we are used to criticizing ourselves for everything we think we are not doing perfectly. I have often heard people on a diet say that they "feel left out" if they are sitting at a table where others are eating something they feel they can't have. It is not surprising because ever since ancient times people have shared meals. If you want to balance your way of eating, it is valuable to be aware of how your need for community affects you.

There is dietary advice suggesting that you should eat by yourself to have more control over what you choose. There are also people that warn of eating alone, stating that this will make it easier to lose control. Some of us "comfort eat" or "wind down" with the help of eating. Often this takes place in solitude and often leads to feelings of shame. For others, eating is just a pleasure.

When it comes to my eating, the human needs I have benefited greatly from exploring are those of belonging, community, meaning, relaxation and autonomy. One way to get to know them is through the feelings we experience when these needs are met and when they are not. Feelings, for example, loneliness or emptiness, can sometimes be misinterpreted as hunger. Read more about emotional hunger on page 42.

Why Do We Eat?

We eat because we need to in order to survive. We eat because of hunger or because a lack of energy tells us that now this organism needs energy and nutrition. We eat to enjoy the experience we get when our senses are stimulated. Many of us eat because it makes it easier to experience community and meaning.

We eat to have fun or to at least avoid feeling bored. We eat to get away from stress, to expe¬rience peace and serenity. We eat because we yearn for comfort or understanding. We eat in moments when we feel lonely and long for warmth and love. We eat because we have told ourselves that we should resist it, and then eating despite this gives us a sense of freedom (at least for a short while). We yearn for freedom and are looking for it in the bottom of the chip bag. Only to be disappointed in the next moment, because once again we have lost control.

People have always shared meals. Food has at all times and in all cultures been a meeting point for people to share food and other joys. Meals have been a gathering point and often they have been followed by dance, music and conversation. Therefore it is not strange if some of us want to eat in order to numb the feelings of loneliness.

When we eat to meet needs other than nutrition and energy, there are often "hidden costs". Maybe we eat things we do not feel good eating, because "it is what is being served". Then we might gain weight, become bored, irritated, stressed or dissatisfied.

If we, on the other hand, sacrifice the need for community in order to experience control over what we eat, it is also costly. Besides our relationships suffering we often experience our world shrinking, instead of gaining a larger sense of freedom and choice. If our eating is regulated by control, instead of natural feelings of hunger and satiety, we more easily become obsessed about food instead of experiencing eating as uncomplicated and natural. Our inner critic grows within us, and our inner peace recedes.

Needbased Eating
Liv Larsson

Certainly we may at times choose to eat alone to better choose when and what we want to eat, but to get caught up in the idea that we cannot eat together with others is too high a price to pay.

If I'm in balance, have the needs like love and belonging met, it is usually the needs of enjoyment, health and energy that I want to meet with eating. If I'm out of balance or feel lonely, it is like there is no bottom to me. Food then becomes love and belonging, but, no matter how much I eat, the "hunger" is still there, craving for more.
-Rachid

A Natural Way of Eating?

If we discover that we are comfort eating in certain situations, we might call a friend instead of adding chocolate sauce to our ice cream.

It can be a gift to yourself to try something new and exciting just for the pleasure of it, rather than to be in continual tight control of what you can eat.

As long as we experience demands around food and weight, we really only have two choices. Either to rebel, which creates resistance or callousness, and often-painful setbacks, or to sub¬mit and agree to do things we do not like, which creates disconnection, lack of autonomy, and in the long run might even flip over into rebellion.

People around the world have repeatedly shown that they are prepared to die in order to ex¬perience freedom. We humans are simply not good slave material. Demanding of ourselves what we should eat and what we should not eat, doesn't consider that we are freedom-loving beings. Our autonomy need will make itself known if we are trying to use coercion on others or ourselves and it might lead to rebellion including eating even more of what we are telling ourselves that we must not eat.

When I tried to find a balanced way to manage my emotional eating, I read the book Fat is a Feminist Issue (1978). When I read it in the mid 80s, it was not a new book, but it is relevant even today (and has been republished many times, the latest being in 2006). One piece of advice from the author that I greatly benefited from was to observe what was going on inside of me when I left anything on the plate.

I realized that I often felt guilt or shame at the bare thought of leaving anything uneaten. I'd rather take another bite for "the starving children in Africa". Early in life I had been taught the importance of "eating everything up" and to not leave anything that I had been served on the plate.

It was neither hunger nor I who decided when I had had enough. The food on the plate was in control. I began consciously to leave something behind at every meal. This made me more aware of how much food I actually put on my plate and taught me about the relationship between my portions and my hunger.

I still agonize over throwing away food I've chosen not to eat. Now my agony is more based on the sadness of wasting food and not on moralizing points. I do not like to throw food away, as I know that resources like food are unevenly distributed in this world. When at times I, with despair, read about how much food is thrown away, it becomes even more important for me to try to contribute to finding ways that we can make friends with our eating habits and with food.

A compilation of four guidelines that has inspired me comes from the book *I Can Make You Thin* by Paul McKenna.

1. Eat when you are hungry.
2. Eat what you want to eat.
3. Enjoy what you are eating.
4. Stop eating when you are full, or if you are not enjoying what you are eating anymore, or when you are not feeling hungry.

These four suggestions are interconnected and build on each other. Their main advantage is not that they can help us find

12

a balanced weight. Why I like them is because they focus on the collaboration between the body and our nature, rather than controlling it. They also embrace the idea that we have a deep need of freedom. This is something that I have often found is lacking in many diets and health remedies. They have a more mechanical approach, telling us what to eat or refrain from eating. This might be helpful for some time, but it does not teach us how to live with a balanced approach to food and our bodies.

When we follow these suggestions, it is common to encounter internal resistance as we have learnt things that are not in line with it. The fourth suggestion supports the experience of feeling free to leave food on the plate and to not stuff ourselves, in order to be polite or to avoid feeling guilty.

Several experiments have been conducted in order to find out how having learned to "eat up all that is on our plate" affects us. In one of the experiments two holes were drilled in a table top in a cafeteria. Over the holes plates were mounted and through tubes placed into the holes more soup could be added to the soup bowls without the test subjects noticing it. The subjects were told that it was the quality of the food that they were there to test.

People who ate from the bowls that were added to, ate 73 % more than those who did not receive any additional soup in their bowls.

Maybe we are driven more than we think by ideas that it is impolite to leave food and that one should eat as much as possible whenever it is available. In any case, it seems that our learned ideas have a major impact on how we deal with our natural satiety. Let's look into the four suggestions a bit deeper.

1. Eat When You are Hungry

Our body is created with a built-in instruction manual. In a sophisticated way we get signals in the form of hunger that tells us that we need food. We feel tired when we need rest or energy. We feel sad when we need to mourn, alone when we need community and bored when we need to experience more stimulation or meaning.

These are signals that newborn children instinctively interpret and act on. Many of us adults have lost touch with these natural signals. The connections between what we feel and what we need is not as clear anymore. We've learned all kinds of things about weight, about how we should look, about food, about what is good or not healthy to eat.

Our thoughts about what we should or should not do clouds our clarity and gets in the way of the innate signals. Eating when you are hungry is one way to re-establish connection with the intrinsic wisdom of the body.

For some it is a challenge to distinguish between emotional and physical hunger. We have received so many messages about what to eat, when we shall eat it, what not to eat, how we should look and weigh, that we are distracted when we are asked to let our natural physical hunger control our choices.

When we don't eat when we are hungry our body lowers the burning of calories. Our body has a super clever survival mechanism, so it makes sure to store energy if we do not eat when we are hungry.

An invaluable step if you want to eat in a natural way is to learn to recognize physical hunger and fullness. If you recognize that this sometimes is a challenge for you, I suggest you use the exercises for week 1 and 2 in the program in this book and the "hunger and satiety scale" on page 40 as long as needed to get more awareness around hunger and eating.

There was a period when I pushed myself to my limit in order to finish a project, and slept very little. It led to a situation where I was often very tired but I did not really want to accept it. My body signaled that it wanted energy. The feeling was fatigue and I tried to fix it with more food or sweets.

The need for rest and sleep "gave up" its natural signals and my tired body tried to find energy in some other way. When I realized I was misinterpreting the feeling of tiredness as hunger, I decided to check in with my need for rest when I was craving sweets, asking myself if I were actually tired and needing to sleep. This led me to rest often for 10 to 15 minutes instead of putting something sweet in my mouth and the sweet craving almost always passed away. Later I read studies that showed that people who sleep less than six hours per day may increase levels of a hormone that increases appetite, especially for calorie rich foods and I guess that was part of what I was going through.

Several of the people that I have guided through the jungle of eating abuse have described that they almost panic when they feel hunger. Or they feel stress and immediately want to get rid of the feeling. To know and accept what hunger feels like, usually calms us. Additionally, embracing the hunger signal provides greater freedom to choose what and when you want to eat.

If you are worried about not being sufficiently full, remind yourself that if you feel hungry again as soon as in 15 minutes, then you can eat more. If you have tried to lose weight and have been practicing repressing feelings of hunger for a long time, this may feel very uncomfortable. At least it was for me. I made it into a challenge to pay attention to the first signals of hunger and to take them "seriously" as I just wanted to escape the intensity they usually brought with them.

If we don't eat when we are hungry, our body's metabolism changes and we burn fewer calories. Basically the body thinks we are under threat of starving and as a super clever survival mechanism, it makes sure we are storing energy.

Become More Aware of Hunger and Fullness

1. Start by studying the scale on page 40. Choose a time and put a number representing where on the hunger scale you are every thirty minutes. Do this at two or three different times in a week.

2. If you find that you don't know if you are hungry or thirsty, start by drinking a glass of water and feel what the signal from your body says.

2. Eat What You Want to Eat

I trust that my body has a natural attraction to the nutrition it needs. There have been several studies in which children during a week or a month received unlimited access to different types of food. All the studies show that over the course of a week, the children have received the nutrition they need.

Our bodies know what they need and try to tell us this. As children, most of us have this connection with the needs of the body intact, but over the years, we unfortunately lose it (or maybe forget it). It seems that it is possible to trust that when our body needs something, it enjoys it more.

From the time my son was two years old, until he was six, I never ceased to be surprised that while he literally shoveled in one type of food on one day, he might reject the same food the next day. I guess his body signaled to him what he needed and he listened to it instead of getting stuck in the idea that he liked or did not like certain foods.

Many of us don't give ourselves the pleasure of truly tasting and enjoying what we eat. We eat what we know feels secure, even though we don't always like the effects it has on our bodies. If you recognize yourself in this, I want to challenge you. During one week, make as many conscious choices as possible about what you eat. Before putting anything in your mouth, ask your body if this is something it longs for.

Also ask after the first, second and third bite if you want to continue. If possible, refrain from what the body doesn't want, whether it is spinach, candy or fruit. Never mind if you have learned that something is unhealthy or healthy. Remember this is an experiment, meant to learn something from.

Eat what you want and let your body guide your choices. When you eat, enjoy it and become alert to your body and your senses. Then stop eating when you feel a satiety signal or are not hungry anymore. People's desire for freedom makes them rebel and eat more of what they see as "forbidden".

When I've talked about how we can trust our inner signals I

have sometimes been met with an horrified exclamation:

"Then I would only eat sweets or junk food!"

But if you also decide to enjoy what you eat and stop eating when you are not hungry anymore, I don't think you need to be worried about this. I have trouble imagining myself fully enjoying something that doesn't make me feel good or that I am allergic to. But if it is potato chips (or something you think is unhealthy) and you are craving that the next time you're hungry, why not try it? Pour the chips into a bowl, and get in touch with your hunger so you can enjoy them. Please try out what I'm suggesting in this book my, but do not continue it if it does not work for you.

The first time I had that kind of craving when I explore this approach to eating I followed this procedure and noticed by the third piece that I was having a hard time fully enjoying what I ate. My enjoyment was disrupted by the fact that I actually wanted to eat something that gave me more energy and nutrition. So I simply switched from the chips to something else that I then focused on enjoying.

For you it might happen faster or you may eat chips for some time. Just make sure to enjoy them! When you are full, you simply stop and the next time you are hungry you connect once again with what you want to chose to eat.

Remember that what I am proposing is not any controlled quick cure or diet. This is a learning process on how to live more in touch with your human needs. I want to support you in finding balanced eating that will last a lifetime.

During a period when I explored this way of eating, I on one occasion, had breakfast at a hotel. I asked myself what I wanted to eat and realized that what I most longed for was to eat a sandwich with marmalade. Instantly two censoring thoughts appeared. One was that it was not healthy and the second was that I had never been particularly fond of marmalade. But this particular morning it was what I was longing for. There was strawberry marmalade and apricot marmalade.

I have never liked apricot marmalade I thought. Once again

I caught myself and asked my body what it really wanted and to my surprise it was the apricot marmalade! I made my sandwich and to my surprise I enjoyed it tremendously and felt very good for the rest of the day. Dried apricots after this often became my choice of a snack and it was not until later that I found out that I had an iron deficiency. Apricots are a good source of iron.

3. Enjoy What you Choose to Eat

Tastes and smells are a natural part of life. Sometimes I play with the idea that we have a certain taste or enjoyment quota to be met for us to feel satisfied. As if nature speaks to us through our senses and makes sure that we get the nutrition we need.

Something that is intimately linked to eating what you want to eat, is that you take the time to enjoy what you choose. To really take the time to experience visuals, smells, and tastes. To allow all the senses to be active when we eat helps us enjoy the food even more.

I have often heard people talk about how they long to eat something special. To my wonderment we eat (yes I write "we" because I've also seen myself doing this) what we longed for, while reading a newspaper or watching TV. We are seemingly totally oblivious that we are eating and how can we then derive any pleasure from our eating. And who has not marveled about how quickly the candy or the snacks ran out, after we have been eating them in front the TV set. Even though you have eaten everything the "enjoyment quota" is not filled and it is easy to want more.

I had difficulties over a period really enjoying whatever I chose to eat. It had been quite easy to learn to choose to eat when I was hungry and quite easy to quit eating when I was full. But I still had a hard time to fully enjoy what I ate.

Before I got used to it, the feeling of freedom was lost by the fact that I was so focused on being aware of the moment when I would be full. I also made various attempts to not do something else when I ate. To not distract myself from the experience of enjoying my food by reading, watching TV or speaking.

But I wriggled like a worm. The agony grew at the thought of not getting to read, watch a movie or talk to someone while I ate and I often didn't last for more than half a meal before I gave in to the urge to do something more than just eat. Additionally, I was so busy NOT doing anything else that I did not enjoy the food at all. I had an idea about how enjoying food meant gluttony, or at least overeating. The fear was that the pleasure would "take over" and that I would not be able to stop myself. At the same time I remembered years of overeating and that it had not at all been enjoyment at the center of the experience then.

As far as I can remember, for five meals in a row I had been eating and been fully concentrated on the experience of eating and not enjoying it. Now I became more curious in exploring this in a different way, where I would not put pressure on myself or force myself to enjoy what I ate (as if that would have been possible under pressure or coercion).

I decided to try it for three meals to give the enjoyment a chance and see what it would bring. What happened was the exact opposite of my assumption, that if I enjoyed the food I would begin gluttonizing. On the contrary, I discovered that when I really focused on enjoying the food, I noticed the very first signals that I was full and could easily stop eating.

A little apprehensive, I was nevertheless about to stop eating something I enjoyed. Then I reminded myself that I could eat again whenever I became hungry and the uneasiness was released. It was as if I fed myself with a new way of thinking. Maybe you would like to try for a short time to focus on enjoying your food, for example by eating in silence or by putting down the cutlery between each bite. Lowering the tempo and enjoying. Not as a "should", but as a game and an experience. To be able to know that we are eating what we want, we need to pay attention to how what we eat tastes. It lays the foundation to understanding the signals that we are getting full.

A Warning and a Suggestion

There are substances in many snacks, such as sugar or glutamate, which are addictive. This makes it difficult to stop eating some snacks, even though one is full. If these kinds of things are what you long for, I have a suggestion. Pour the amount of chips or candy you think you want to eat in a bowl and set aside the rest. Then simply eat and enjoy what you have set aside to eat. When you have eaten whatever is in the bowl, ask yourself if you are still hungry and if you are enjoying what you are eating. If the answer is yes, refill and continue to enjoy.

4. Stop Eating When You no Longer are Enjoying What You are Eating, are Full or Don't Feel Hunger

"How do I know when to stop eating?" is a common question I get when I talk about this fourth suggestion. Fullness is not as clear as hunger. It has a delayed signal so we can benefit greatly from learning to recognize the first signs of being full.

There is all sorts of advice about how to eat until you are 80% full or to eat for a maximum of 30 minutes and at least eat for 15 minutes. This has to do with the fact that it can take up to 20 minutes for the signals from the stomach to reach the brain leaving the message that we are now full.

The above suggestions can be valuable, but there are other ways to handle this challenge. I have greater confidence that we are creating more balance in our eating when we base our choices on the signals from our body, rather than on any other method.

We can sharpen our ability to decide when we are full by getting to know the different signs of being full. Hunger is persistent and determined. It aches and rips inside us to be sure that we act. The feelings of hunger bangs on our door until we listen and give the body what it needs. Hunger is an excellent signal for the initiation of a meal, but to know when it is time to stop, we also need to understand the many aspects of fullness. Satiety is blunter than hunger and arrives with some delay. It increases gradually so that when we are eating something, it takes a while for the body to register and signal that we've had enough. We can learn to pay attention to the more subtle signals that we have actually had enough to make sure we stop in time.

The old saying "hunger is the best spice" holds great truth. The simplest meal can taste heavenly when we are hungry. And even the most delicious meal tastes, after a certain number of bites not as tasty anymore. When the food doesn't taste as good, this is a first signal from the body that it is starting to get full. That signal comes before you feel full.

To draw attention to the subtle inner messages, we need to pay attention to what's going on in our body and in our minds. Enjoying the food lays the foundation for us to catch when it is time to stop eating as well.

If we eat while we are reading, watching TV or doing anything else that distracts us, it is easy to miss the first signals of fullness[3]. The flavors and the smells are not as clear to us when we are busy with other things and we run the risk of eating more than we later enjoy.

When I went through treatment for my unbalanced way of eating, I was very confused about how a natural way of eating could even look. With the support of my therapist I decided that for a start my meals would not be shorter than 15 minutes and no longer than 30 minutes.

When 10 minutes had passed I asked myself after every bite if I needed more food. I thereby became more aware of the body's signals and when I was becoming full. It took me out of my habitual eating, but I still had a long way to go to totally calibrate my system so that I could follow my internal clock, rather than an external one.

---

3 For suggestions on practicing the ability to become more aware of hunger signals see page 41.

Gluttony

For millions of years we lived as gatherers. As gatherers we walked long distances every day to made sure we had food for our group. The group shared the food available with each other, and in that way everyone received food - even the young, the old and the sick. To share became a survival strategy even if it meant that one ate very little for long periods of time.

When at times someone found plenty of food that was greasy or sweet one turned to gluttony - also a survival strategy. Everyone filled their fat reserves, to be used for times when there was not as much food. In this way, one can argue that gluttony is a naturally inherited survival impulse. When I read Lasse Berg describe this in his book, Dawn over the Kalahari: how humans became human, I felt a great relief. The shame that I had felt all my life about eating "too much" changed.

It reminded me of how different it felt for me to eat to numb emotional hunger than when I ate for other reasons. It can feel different on different occasions. I can feel guilt and remorse over the fact that I gulped down a few extra sandwiches in solitude one evening when I had previously made up my mind to go on a diet and lose weight. A common sign that we have eaten out of emotional hunger is that we feel guilt or shame afterwards.

On another occasion I have gone to bed stuffed after a completely wonderfully delightful dinner with friends, where we tasted food from different parts of the world. Although I ate without being hungry and was already full, I was not doing it to push away shame or some other uncomfortable feeling, but to have fun. I had eaten because I was curious and sharing an adventure together with good friends. It was obvious to me that I had done it because I had chosen it and not as a rebellion against inner demands.

But one question remains - how can we manage ancient impulses to gluttony in a society where we live in abundance? Where we can go into a supermarket and are exposed to more food in ten minutes than what we would only have seen 1000 years ago over several months. How can we make life-serving choices in that situation? There are no simple answers to the question. What I know is that it usually only makes me feel worse if I blame myself after having stuffed myself.

In any case it doesn't make any difference in the long run as I do not learn anything new if I only blame myself for old mistakes.

If you overeat, I have two pieces of advice to give you, (and please only read them if you want any advice at the moment): One is to talk to others about it; others that will not increase your shame and guilt but rather listen to you and together with you try to find new ways to manage your eating. The second is to use the tools from page 38 and onwards for some time and see if it makes any difference for you.

Your Food & Eating History

When I was small and got bored, I whiningly used to tell my mom, "I'm bored; I can't think of anything fun to do?". She was often busy and I quickly learnt that the stress she felt in this situation made it easy to get her to give me some money to buy some sweets. It gave me a moment of meaning, and yes even a sense of belonging. It became "My candy and I" and I felt less lonely and bored.

As an adult, I have rarely eaten to comfort myself when I feel sad. Significantly, more often I've eaten when I've felt restless. I connect this to that early-learned strategy of eating to drive away a sense of boredom. I've had to work to obtain more awareness in managing my need for meaning and consciously choosing something that is truly satisfying.

Many people I've talked to recognize themselves in this, but also in consoling themselves by eating when they feel sad. How many of us received an offer of something sweet to console us when we were small and sad or cried.

I suggest that many of us have learned to eat when we have

felt something, which was actually linked to some other need than for energy. It might be the need for stimulation, meaning, belonging, or to be understood. This insight was empowering for me because it means it is possible to learn new strategies.

The first step is to teach myself to recognize what I feel and need. When I understand what my need is, I can make more conscious choices. I can choose to eat or do something else, for example, to experience meaning and stimulation.

> Reflecting on one's eating history provide valuable clues as to what affects one's eating. How did you talk about food and weight in your family of origin? How, what and when did you eat? What space did feelings get? How did you take care of the needs for autonomy, community, empathy and meaning?

Thin = Happy?

Although this book is about something as private as eating, I can not help but write a few lines about how the pursuit of being thin connects with the way our society functions. For over 20 years I have thought that if only I could get thin enough I would be happy. That if only I could become thin, I would forever soar on pink clouds. Furthermore, "the thinner, the better" has felt true for many years.

These thoughts were part of why I starved myself for years and for more years binged and vomited. This was over an extreme period of eight years that started in my teens.

Now I know better, but have also realized that these learned beliefs are something I will probably live with all my life. My Mom, who is 78, remains concerned that she is fat, not for health reasons but for appearance, so it doesn't seem to disappear with age either.

Even though men also feel pressure to be thin, women's pursuit of beauty and slenderness seems to have lost any proportion of sanity. A woman's main competitive advantage has been for ages and in many cultures her appearance. A beautiful woman

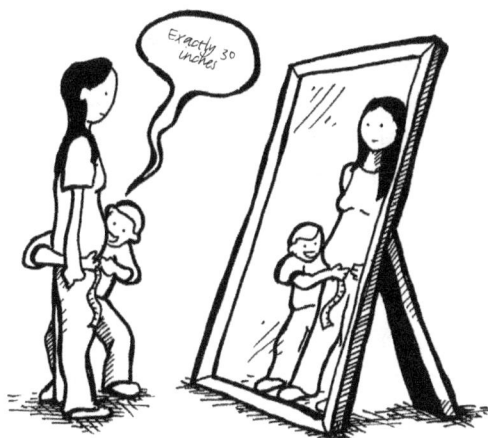

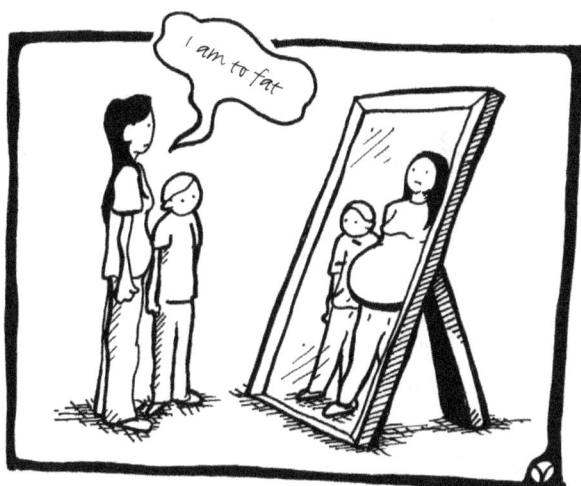

can get a man who has power, and thus gain access to some power herself. Women's striving to live up to the prevailing ideals of beauty has created powerlessness at the same time. So much of women's power is focused on this one thing: to become thin and beautiful. We go from one diet or treatment after another and who has the energy to care about how power is divided in society or inequities if one is exhausted by the latest diet.

We are tremendously easy to manipulate if we're kept captive in dissatisfaction with our bodies. If a woman can't be kept in her place in some other way, then why not pump her full of messages such as "a beautiful woman is a slender woman".

Even thin underwear models are retouched so that we get

strange ideas of how a woman's body should look – the representations often don't match reality.

On the website "43Things," users can add a list of their life goals. Losing weight is the most common goal. Although that partially reflects the daily thoughts moving within people than actual life goals, it does say something about what impact these thoughts have on us.

Research does not support the idea that if we were thinner, we would be happier[4].

Becoming thin may give us a fleeting sense of happiness, but it doesn't last. After a while the level of happiness goes down again. Yet many of us long for it, trusting that it will really make us happy.

The Freedom Struggle of The Slimmer

Of course you have to eat your delicious porridge.
Because if you don't eat your delicious porridge, then
You can't grow big and strong. And if
you don't grow big and strong, you will not have the energy to
force your kids when you get some, to eat
their delicious porridge.
Astrid Lindgren through Pippi Longstocking, 1948.

The inner struggle of the slimmer is a freedom struggle. Their freedom is threatened by the rigorous diet one has set up and which shall be followed to the letter. Many have noticed the negative impact that "should" has on the motivation for physical exercise. It has never been as comfortable to remain in bed as when we have decided to begin a new exercise program that morning. We twist and turn in order to experience freedom, but can't find it in bed, nor in the forced exercise round.

---

4 Lyubomirsky, Sonja (2008), The How of Happiness: A Scientific Ap¬proach to getting the life you want.

Often we violate the rules, although we ourselves have set them up, in our search for more freedom. And when we finally feel free, this is followed by disappointment, because behind the schedule we were determined to follow was a whole series of needs, for example, hope, health, beauty, community and meaning, which are now not being met. So if we want to manage our eating in a way that works for us in the long run, we need to see the need for freedom as part of our nature. We need to bring that aspect into the equation as well and make sure we experience autonomy. When we approach food with the thoughts – "I can not eat this because I need to lose weight" or "I should eat healthier," it will make it more difficult for us to achieve our goals. When we eat something because we think we deserve it, it may also get in the way of our goals and our connection with ourselves. Usage of rewards as well as punishment is a system meant to control slaves, not a way to motivate free people.

Health and self-love don't grow under coercion. They grow if we give ourselves what we need, and remember that the need for freedom is part of our human nature. Susanne, a woman I tutored in her eating, began to lose weight and noticed a strong emotion that she could not understand. She weighed about 15 kg more than she wanted to and had pain in both her knees and hips. For many years, she had tried to find balance between food and weight, but had not succeeded with the help of any of the many diets she had attempted. The third time we met she had discovered something that was a turning point for her.

Susanne realized that this certain feeling always crept up on her every time she had lost some weight. As long as she could remember a vague fear came over her without any obvious reason. She had often started to binge on these occasions, until finally she was back to the weight she had been before she started to lose. Then the binging would fade away (or she would binge out of sadness and hopelessness at having gained weight once again).

Now she connected to a memory from when she was a child and had been forced to eat during a period when she was sick.

Her mother was frightened, as Susanne had become very thin, and forced her to eat. She had put food on Susanne's plate and did not let her leave the table until she had finished all of it.

Now she saw the connection between the feeling that came over her when she had lost weight and the memory of her mother's worry. She connected to the sadness and realized that her need for respect and autonomy had not been met at those times of being forced to eat. When she got in touch with these needs she could start to choose more consciously when and what she ate. It also became important for her to listen to her body for what it wanted, and not only to what she had taught herself was healthy or appropriate. She found a way to cooperate with her body and to find a path to true health and wellbeing. It was when she ate with the need for respect, autonomy and health that she started to find a balanced way of eating.

Internal and External Body Images

If I had been a model for the Swedish painters Carl Larsson or Anders Zorn, from the start of the 20th century, I might have perceived myself as beautiful. My body is suited for the cultural ideals of beauty in those days. But after browsing contemporary magazines, my inner critic often gets so much nutrition that it goes wild.

In these magazines there is often advice on how to lose weight, get a flatter stomach, bigger or smaller muscles and about what one should and shouldn't eat. I often feel more worried and self-conscious after reading a magazine like this, and find my inner critic is nagging me about loosing weight. Rigorously controlled food schedules, lists of what food one should buy and eat, as well as what not to buy or eat, makes the reading feel as if one is in a war zone where every little action needs to be checked and controlled so as not to cause more danger.

Change

Many of us have learned that change comes when we use appropriate rewards and punishments. We punish someone when they have done something we think is bad and hope they will learn from the punishment and never do it again. We reward someone when they have done what we think of as right or appropriate and hope that this will make them continue such behavior. But if we want to create behavioral changes that persist, something completely different than punishments and rewards are needed. Punishments and rewards create short term and externally controlled actions. I am looking to create change that leads to a more lasting balance in an experience of freedom.

When we are connected to ourselves at the level of needs, deep change may happen. When we are in touch with what we need, we can choose more satisfying ways to meet our needs. Compassion and self-empathy are great support in order to be able to do this internal change. Self-empathy is about getting in touch with what is going on within you and embracing it, whatever it is.

Change occurs suddenly or over time when we accept life from within. But it is only after some time that we can see if that which we changed will lead to something stable. Sometimes, we don't succeed with something we have set out for ourselves and we start blaming ourselves.

If we have tried to motivate change, even for the better, with telling ourselves that we should or must do something, we are likely to get more judgmental of ourselves if we fail to live up to our goals.

It is difficult to change when we are in the middle of a full-blown self-criticism attack. All our energy goes into defending ourselves from more pain. All our energy goes to defend ourselves from more pain. It is easy to start thinking that "there is something wrong with the desired change or with us", so we might just as well give up on any change for the better because "we do not deserve it" or will "never be able to live up to our goal". In order to gain the strength to move on, it is useful to instead get more deeply connected with the needs we tried to meet with changing something in our lives. Getting connected to what motivates us to keep working for our goal can help us overcome obstacles on the way.

We can also gain clarity on our resistance by connecting to the needs that are not being met by what we have set up to do. Maybe that which we had planned, without us being aware of it, had too high a price for our need for community. Or maybe your need for autonomy will be knocking on your door if you try to change with the help of the coercive "must change" or "should change".

Connect to the needs you tried to meet by not doing what you had in mind. After that you might want to change something about the way you make the changes you want to see in your life.

This time choose a strategy that has the potential to also embrace the needs that were not being met by the first way you chose.

Can This Ever Change

To break habits around eating and relating to one's body in new ways is often a challenge. In the beginning new choices can take tremendous effort. Regardless if we have an iron will or not, many of us fall back into old comfortable habits when we are exposed to stress of any kind. "You just have to make up your mind" is correct to some degree, but change takes more than that.

Learning new things can sometimes seem difficult. Sometimes we think that we are making progress and sometimes we think we are standing still. Learning is a process in which we constantly take small or big steps, not really knowing beforehand how it will proceed.

The ladder of competnece is a model to illustrate how change occurs. The first step symbolizes being unaware of what it is we

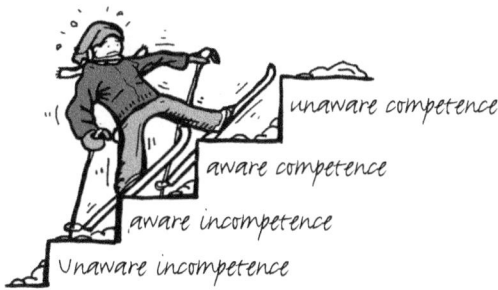

unaware competence
aware competence
aware incompetence
unaware incompetence

do not know. On this step, we are not aware that we want to change or can develop. Something needs to happen for us to realize it.

Perhaps in reading this book so far, you have taken a step up to the next step of conscious incompetence. Here we understand that we may find it useful to learn something and we may deliberately seek information or to develop support. Patience is now needed to put up with "feeling stupid and incompetent." When we then learn something, we can take another step up - to conscious competence. We see how our new knowledge can be used, but it can still take quite an effort to make new choices. We might rebel or give up when we think that we can no longer blame the fact that we don't know how to progress.

Once we get over the rebel phase, we can take advantage of our knowledge and we are now ready for the next step. It's called unaware competence. Here we have managed to create a routine, habit or automatic reaction in which we use our knowledge unconsciously. We don't need to make an effort or look for the knowledge because it's already there.

> To exercise your ability for self-empathy:
> Connect inwardly, as often as you remember to, by asking yourself:
>
> - What do I feel right now?
> - What do I need right now?

Presence

To draw attention to emotions and body signals, we need to have presence. When we have presence it is so much easier to make conscious choices. It is also easier to enjoy what we are eating and to use the tools I describe later in this book.

> I eat only to maintain this body
> not for intoxication, not for play
> not for beauty
> not for pleasure, not for pain.

The above words are from the grace we read before our meals in a ten-day meditation retreat in a Thai monastery I once attended. It was a way to focus on the central need to eat and to open our hearts to what we received, with gratitude.

It has come back to me many times, when I've focused on other needs for my eating such as belonging and meaning. Next time you eat something and at the same time feel hesitant, maybe because of thoughts that tell you that you "shouldn't" or "must not" eat this, remind yourself that a fundamental purpose of eating is to keep your physical body alive. Ask yourself, with gentle care, if this need is included in your choice to eat right now. It tends to make it easier to choose if you are connected to this.

There are many different ways of saying grace at the table, from different traditions and religions. Maybe you want to try one of them for a time, or write your own. Or maybe it would suit you better to just sit in silence for a short while before you eat or to say something to the people you are sharing the meal with.

In many traditions, cultures and religions it is usual to say grace or "break bread" in some form. It often includes gratitude but also remembering how things are interconnected, how come we have been given this food and where it comes from. It is often about thanking a source of all life as well.

While working with the different exercises in the book, many of the people that tried them out became connected with a strong desire to be more aware before they ate something. Many just ate and it was only when they became too full, that they remembered that they had wanted to stop and connect to the needs they wanted to meet in their eating.

Perhaps saying grace has a greater potential than just making us aware of what we are grateful about. Perhaps a moment of stillness at the beginning of the meal becomes the moment of connection that is necessary for us to choose more consciously, experiencing our hunger. It may help us to become still enough to be able to pay attention to the signals when we have had enough and let the body decide when it's time to eat and not to eat.

To be aware of how I sit when I eat has also helped me to be more present to the signals. I noticed at one point that I was sitting in a certain way when I ate. Either I put my legs crossed or sat on them. So out of curiosity I decided to explore what would happen if I sat with both legs straight down next to each other.

It was really difficult at first. Time after time I discovered that I had crossed my legs. To sit with my feet on the floor made me restless and the legs vibrated with nervous energy. My way of eating was changed by getting to know this intensity. It increased my attention and made me more aware of how things tasted, helped me to enjoy it as it was and to stop when it no longer tasted as good or when my stomach felt full. The whole experience became very intense and also interesting.

When in the 80s I took part in a number of meditation retreats - based on Vipassana Buddhist meditation - in Asia, "Mindfulness training" was an important part. During one occasion, we were served a little bit of mango. The task was to watch it in silence and become aware of one's reactions, then take it in your hand, put it into your mouth, suck it, feel the texture, notice the taste, chew slowly and feel how it felt inside your mouth before swallowing it. It became an almost holy moment, where all the senses were affected. Gratitude and wonder aroused in a way that I often try to remind myself of, even when I eat "fast food".

Many people have said that they have gained insight into how they eat by regularly writing some kind of food diary. There are a number of Internet-based applications that help to keep track of calorie content.

I have mixed feelings around this. One is I really feel hope, seeing the difference it can make. When we write down everything we eat, it is difficult to close our eyes to how our intake really looks. It gives clarity on what we can change if we want to affect our health and weight.

I have also heard people say that once they stopped writing, they lost awareness of this again. They then started to eat much larger quantities in a kind of rebellion. Probably their writing was more about control than about laying the foundations for cooperating with the body.

So if it brings a sense of clarity and presence to write a food diary, I think it's a great help. But I believe that it has to be done with a certain attitude and curiosity. If it becomes a kind of controlling surveillance, perhaps you would be better off doing something else to create more awareness of what and why you are eating.

Another method that has been valuable to me in this exploration is HeartMath.[5] This method is simple and is based on a breathing exercise. Simplified, one can say that the intention is to create coherence between the heart and the brain. It seems to help some people to find new ways to have less stress and tension around their eating habits.

---

5 Read more about HeartMath on www.heartmath.org

Eating Consciously - exercise

Do this exercise[6] if you want to hone your ability to enjoy what you eat and be present with what's going on inside of you when you do it. Pay attention to the critical or judgmental thoughts that come up, note them and then let them go. Focus on observing. Pay attention to how your senses are stimulated, without evaluating the experience as good or bad.

Allow yourself to play with the idea that you're an alien that has fallen into a human body and eats for the first time. For the exercise you need one apple or some other fruit per day for seven days. Start by selecting an apple. If you have two apples you look at them, and choose the one you feel most attracted to. If you are in a store you might have hundreds of apples to choose from. Give yourself some time to choose and pay attention to how it feels.

The next step, perhaps when you're at home, or have peace and quiet around you, is to focus on the fact that you soon are about to eat the apple. Take a small pause. Do you feel the body beginning to prepare?

If you're hungry, maybe the saliva is flowing and the stomach is purring. Or maybe there is no reaction. Just notice what's happening without trying to change any judgments that come up. Now take a bite of the apple. Be as concentrated as possible on the experience. Be especially observant of your senses.

What do you hear? How does the apple feel in your mouth? Do you observe any scent and taste? Eat the apple and do nothing else for a few minutes. When the apple has been eaten, focus on the experience of just having eaten it. How does the apple affect you now? After a minute? After five minutes?

Eat nothing more for a while, notice if the apple makes you hungry or full. Repeat the exercise once each day for a week.

---

6 Inspired by a mindfulness exercise from Åsa Nilsonne's blog.

Create Balance

To contribute to your exploration of how you relate to food, weight, health and body, I have put together a 12-week program. There is no reason to rush through the exercises, but rather let each part take its time. The 12 weeks is just a suggestion.

Some exercises build on each other but most can be done separately if you want to change their order. Rather use a longer time than a shorter one to take away any sense of pressure. Certain exercises you might want to do for two weeks or longer.

The intention is not to go through a fast diet. It's not about creating rapid changes or helping you to lose weight. However, the exercises might help you to find lasting freedom, relaxation

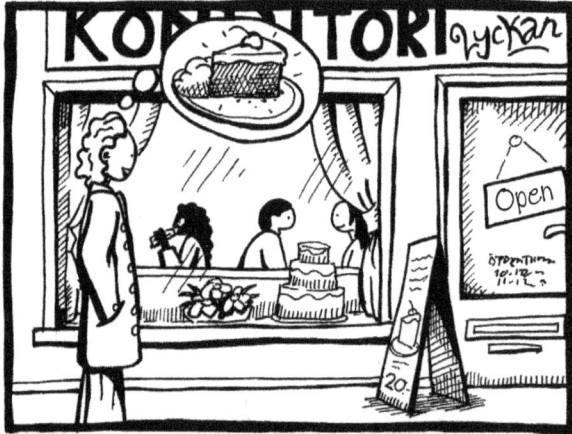

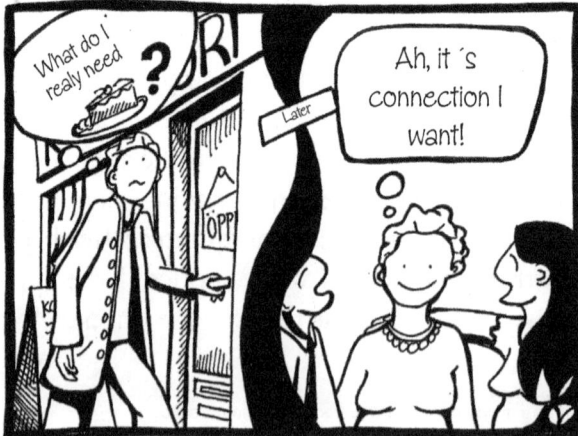

and enjoyment in relation to food and weight. It's also not about fixing yourself or cheering yourself up. With these exercises, you lay a foundation for a balanced cooperation with yourself. It may take some time. Let the changes come from within. Focus on increasing your connection with yourself rather than focusing on bodily changes.

Learn about what is happening in you in relation to eating, food and your body. Let it be a slow process, this is your life. The important thing is what you learn by going through the program, reflecting over the needs you are trying to meet with eating or not eating and in reading the book, not whether or not you can follow everything to the letter. If it becomes a demand there is a risk that you will rebel to find the feeling of freedom again. We are poorly equipped to be slaves.

If possible, play with this training program together with someone else. In that way you get to both give and receive support, which will deepen your learning. If you don't find someone else who wants to do the exercises, maybe you can find someone who is interested in listening to what you learn and give you support in any challenges you face.

Doing these exercises might feel very private at the start but sharing about things we usu-ally hide, with someone we trust can be a big healing in itself. But if the thought of sharing it with someone increases tension around this too much, please make sure you take it easy with yourself.

Ask For Support

When we make changes around our eating our environment often notices it. Reflect on if you have any requests to the people you often eat together with. Maybe you want to tell them that you're looking for more freedom of choice around your eating. Ask them to keep from trying to get you to eat more, less or something else than what you have chosen. Maybe you want to tell them that you want to enjoy what you choose to eat and ask them to keep from making comments about what is healthy or unhealthy on your plate. If you want to try all or part of the exercise program, maybe you want to tell the people immediately around you about it. Ask for the support you would want and need to experiment with it.

The Tool Box

1. Hunger and satiety scale.
2. Knowing emotional and physical hunger.
3. Needs Inventory.

There is a saying - "The road to hell is paved with good intentions" - that can very well be connected to eating. Many of us may recognize the scenario where one day we decide it is now time to deal with healthier eating, only to find ourselves sitting the next day in front of the TV again with a candy bag, our usual snack, or that big bowl of our favorite ice cream.

Coping with one's - perhaps complicated - relationship to food and weight only with the help of will power is virtually impossible. If during a day you have observed your will and how it has followed your emotional waves, you have probably realized that it is a not a too reliable means of support. However, our will is important to trigger our urge to care for our body and our health and to start thinking about how we want to do so.

Two of the tools we will use during the program are the hunger and satiety scale and the chart about emotional and physical hunger.

The hunger and satiety scale has been compiled by Robert Fritz and I borrowed it from the book Eat by choice not by habit, by Sylvia Haskvitz. Haskvitz claims that from a physiological perspective, it is best to eat when you are at 3 or possibly 2 and to stop eating when you are at 5 or 6. She states that if you do this over a period of time, you will end up at a normal weight.

Creating balance and freedom in your eating - 12 Week Exploration

Week 1 - Understanding hunger and satiety

Week 2 – Getting to know fullness

Week 3 - Getting to know hunger

Week 4 – Following four suggestions

Week 5 - What are the needs I am trying to meet by eating?

Week 6 - Are my choices working?

Week 7 - Do I want to choose something new?

Week 8 – Finding Presence with what it means to eat

Week 9 - Finding freedom of choice

Week 10 - Deepening your clarity around hunger and fullness

Week 11 – Finding a natural way of eating

Week 12 - Deepened awareness of hunger and fullness

Tool 1:

Hunger/satiety scale

0. Beyond hungry - feeling weak or going on adrenaline.

1. Too hungry to care about what I eat - Risk of overeating.

2. Very hungry - need to eat now!

3. Moderately hungry - you could wait longer.

4. A little hungry - first thought of food.

5. Neutral - no hunger, no experience of food in the stomach.

6. Satisfaction - feel the food but are not entirely full, no discomfort.

7. Easy discomfort - a little too full, aware of food in the stomach.

8. Discomfort - full, the belly is complaining.

9. Very full - want to lie down to digest food.

10. Tremendously full - so full that it hurts.

The words we use to describe something within us are just words. I have no way of knowing that the words I use to describe how it feels for me when I am full works for you. What you call a three on the scale does not necessarily correspond as the same experience for anyone else. Maybe you want to make your own list, choosing new words. Remember, this is a tool for you to make friends with your inner reactions. Use it as it suits you. I also hope - and I hope this with all my heart – that you do not use these scales to hit yourself with. It might be tempting to do that if you have learned that you get results by punishing or criticizing yourself.

You might be tempted to say things like: "You should have

stopped at number six" or "Now you did it again, no wonder you ate too much when you waited until so long to eat!" I am asking you to use the scale as a frame of reference rather than as a weapon to hurt yourself with. In the following exercises I refer to the numbers in the first scale. But for some people the scale below seems to work better, so feel free to use that one if it fits better for you in your exploration.

Hunger scale 2

1. Almost Fainting

2. Starving

3. Hungry

4. A bit hungry

5. Neutral

6. Full

7. Very full

8. Too full

9. About to burst

10. Nauseous

Tool 2:

Knowing physical and emotional hunger

Physical hunger

- Builds gradually.
- Experienced below the neck.
- Happens (most often) some hours after a meal.
- Disappears when you are full.
- Eating leads to satisfaction.

Emotional hunger

- Appears suddenly.
- Felt above the neck (for example: A craving for potato chips or something sweet).
- Occurs irregularly without direct connection to a given moment.
- Continues even if one eats.
- Eating leads to guilt or shame or discomfort of some other kind.

Being clear about the difference between being physically hungry and emotionally hungry is very valuable. When we are physically hungry and eat, the food provides energy. When we eat when we are emotionally hungry, the food numbs or calms us. This numbing may make us feel calmer, but it might also get in the way of us finding the energy and motivation to meet the needs that were actually there. Many of us mistake, for example, grief, loneliness or emptiness for hunger. That's what I call emotional hunger.

When we cannot distinguish between emotional and physiological hunger, we might choose the strategy to eat, even though there are other strategies that would better meet our needs in these situations, such as seeking out support or empathy from someone we trust. So there is a great benefit in learning to recognize hunger and satiety, but also in learning to recognize anxiety, sadness, restlessness and irritation.

Emotions give us signals about what we need. Because emotions are messengers of something so important, it is useful to have contact with them. If we eat to numb our feelings we might miss information that could help us enjoy our lives even more.

One way to use this tool is to use it directly on the spot, at some point when you're not sure if you are physically hungry or not. Read through the list on page 42 of what characterizes physical hunger and see if you recognize what is going on inside of you.

Ask yourself:
Am I physically hungry?
If the answer is no, ask yourself:
- What are my feelings at this moment?

Listen to the answer and use it to answer the question about what you need right now.
If the answer is, for example, I feel lonely, you might want to seek out someone to talk to or do something else with. If the answer is, I feel restless, perhaps you want to take a walk instead of eating or do both.

Emotional hunger

One of my most clarifying experiences of being emotionally hungry happened on a summer day on my way to meet a friend. It was a 30-minute drive to the beach we had decided to meet on. I had just eaten breakfast when I got into the car. Five minutes from our house I was suddenly hungry. If I had had access to the paragraphs on page 42, I might have realized that the "hunger" came suddenly and not gradually as physical hunger does. If someone had asked me where in the body I felt this hunger, I would not have had an answer, but still I defined what I felt as hunger. Possibly I did wonder about how it had come on so close after eating breakfast, but still now I was hungry, and I felt it. Since I knew I would soon come to a kiosk, I decided to go in and buy a chocolate bar, as that was exactly what I was "hungry" for. When I pulled up in front of the kiosk, I realized that it was Sunday morning and that it had not yet opened.

By the time I met my friend there were tears streaming down my face. My need was to mourn, not to eat. When I had talked with my friend for a while, it became clear where the sadness came from and the thoughts on eating were gone and so was the hunger. Her empathy nurtured me in a much deeper way than one chocolate bar could have ever done. I also gained clarity about some important changes I wanted to make in my life.

When I later read the points on page 42, I recognized what had happened. I both felt wonder and was horrified by how often I had missed moments where I could have received guidance on what I needed.

It also made me more curious to notice and observe situations when I try to suppress feelings. After all, it does not really matter if I weigh 5 kg more or less. But it matters how I feel and if I can enjoy my life.

Tool 3:

Needs Inventory

Before you use the exercise program I suggest that you make an overview of how your needs affect your choices around eating. You will be supported in this overview by having clarity when you use the book and if you do the exercises. I suggest that you do it before week 1 in the program, and also after week 10, and compare the answers to see if anything has changed. Reflect on which of the needs you have attempted to meet by eating over the last few days. Try as much as possible to ignore if you think it was a good or a bad choice. Go through the questions at least three times for a clear overview.

1. During the last few days, have you been trying to meet any of the below needs by eating?

Energy and nutrition? ☐

Freedom and self-determination? ☐

Love and warmth? ☐

Security? ☐

Belonging? ☐

Relaxation? ☐

Inspiration? ☐

Meaning? ☐

Intimacy? ☐

Respect? ☐

Acceptance? ☐

To be seen and heard? ☐

Some other need? ....?

2. Regardless if the needs that motivated you to eat something were met or not, consider more ways to meet them. What could you do, besides eating, to meet these needs?

Belonging:
Example: To take a walk with my friends instead of our usual coffee together.

Belonging:

Meaning:

Freedom and self-determination:

Security:

Inspiration:

Love and warmth:

Intimacy:

Respect:

Acceptance:
To be seen and heard:

Some other need? ....

(Use the list of needs on page 49 for support.)

3. What emotions do you often experience when you are satisfied with what and when you eat? (Use lists of emotions on page 49 as support.)

4. What needs are you trying to meet by eating?

Freedom and self-determination?   ☐

Security?   ☐

Belonging?   ☐

Peace and calmness?   ☐

Inspiration?   ☐

Love and warmth?   ☐

Meaning?   ☐

Intimacy?   ☐

Respect?   ☐

Acceptance?   ☐

To be seen and heard?   ☐

Energy and nutrition?   ☐

Some other need? ....

(Use the list of words for needs on page 49 as support.)

5. What needs are you less satisfied with trying to meet by eating?

Freedom and self-determination? ☐

Security? ☐

Belonging? ☐

Peace and calmness? ☐

Love and warmth? ☐

Meaning? ☐

Intimacy? ☐

Respect? ☐

Acceptance? ☐

To be seen and heard? ☐

Energy and nutrition? ☐

Some other need? ....

(Use the list of needwords on page page 49 as support.)

6. What emotions come up when you are not satisfied with what and when you eat? Use lists of words for emotions on page 49 as support. You might also want to read the paragraph on page 71 about shame.

Words for feelings

Afraid
Alive
Ambivalent
Angry
Ashamed
Awake
Bored
Calm
Comfortable
Confused
Curious
Delighted
Depressed
Desperate
Disappointed
Disinterested
Downhearted

Embarrassed
Energetic
Enthusiastic
Frustrated
Furious
Gloomy
Grateful
Grumpy
Happy
Hopeful
Impatient
Irritated
Lonely
Moved
Nervous
Overwhelmed
Perplexed

Proud
Restless
Sad
Satisfied
Shocked
Skeptical
Stressed
Sure
Surprised
Suspicious
Tense
Thrilled
Tired
Uncomfortable
Uneasy
Upset
Vulnerable
Worried

Words for needs

Acceptance
Acknowledgment
Authenticity
Autonomy
Balance
Beauty
Belonging
Care
Celbration
Choice
Clarity
Closeness
Communication
Community
Connection
Cooperation
Creativity
Ease

Efficiency
Empathy
Equality
Freedom
Fun, Play
Harmony
Health
Honesty
Importance
Inspiration
Integrity
Learning
Light
Love
Meaning
Movement
Mutuality
Nurturance

Order
Participation
Peace
Predictability
Protection
Relaxation
Respect
Rest, sleep
Safety
Sexual expression
Shared reality
Support
To be seen & heard
To contribute
To mourn
Touch
Trust
Understanding
Warmth

The exploration program

Week 1

Learning about hunger and how it feels to be full

1. Where am I right now on the fullness /hunger scale? _____

The focus this week is on increasing your awareness around hunger and fullness. As often as possible during the week, pay attention to where you are on the hunger / fullness scale.
Note which number describes your hunger / fullness level.
I suggest that you keep a "hunger / fullness diary" to note patterns. Maybe there are certain times of the day when you notice hunger, or feel like eating. Write down the number plus a few words about what you feel and think at this time.

Try not to sensor or try to get a "good result". Simply start by noticing the inner signals and how you react to them as much as possible.

Do this on at least three occasions for a clearer picture. Write down the number plus a few words about what you feel and think at this time.

Week 2
Getting to know fullness

1. Where am I right now at the fullness/ hunger scale ____

Some people call being full the absence of hunger, but I think you'll find that it's much more than that. During the first week, you hopefully got an overview of how being hungry or full affects you.

This week's focus is on getting to know what fullness feels like. You will connect deeper with what is happening with your sense of fullness in the end, or after a meal or snack. Don't worry so much about hunger this week, as we will explore it during Week 3.

You can choose a particular day or a particular meal every day when you put an extra focus on satiety. I suggest that you start today or tomorrow. You can also choose to pay attention to your experience of feeling full over a period of time during the day, for example, between one o'clock and four each afternoon. Choose to do this exercise in a way that makes it most likely that you will actually do it. For some people it is a great support to keep some kind of notes or a diary of your insights.

Start by reading through the hunger / satiety scale and the description of emotional and physical hunger on page 42. Support your exploration by writing them down and hang them or in a place where you will see them often.

Take 5 - 10 minutes to notice how it feels to be full. You can be anywhere between 4-9 on the hunger scale. You do not need to stuff yourself to do this.

Ask yourself:

- How do I know that I'm full? Where in the body do I feel it? In the stomach? The neck? Does it feel cold or hot? Is there any movement or is it still? Do I feel heaviness or ease? Energy or fatigue? Do you notice anything else in the body?

What thoughts come with satiety? (Often we have been taught to think in a certain way, which sometimes can be supportive and sometimes may lie in the way. They can, for example, be thoughts of gratitude or thoughts that we should have eaten something else than what we chose.

If this exercise triggers strong emotions that are difficult to handle on your own, you can shorten the time you observe satiety. You can also skip it or adjust it in any way that suits you. Remind yourself that this exercise is not about changing anything, losing weight or controlling yourself, but only about getting to know your own natural impulses better.)

A supplementary tool for this week is to answer these questions. Do it in a way that supports you, it might be every day, a few times a day or every second day.

1. Where am I right now on the satiety / hunger scale? _____

2. Where in my body do I feel it? Describe the feeling and where in the body you experience it.

3. Am I satisfied or dissatisfied with my choices? Do I have an internal pep talk after my meals? Or do I criticize myself for what and how much I have eaten? Am I trying to smooth over something you dislike that I have done?

4. Are there some thoughts that are more usual in moments when I feel full?

5. Which of my needs are often met when I feel full? (use the list of need words on page 49.)

6. Are there any needs that are not met? What emotions are helping you to pay attention to those needs?

I've noticed that I feel safe when I'm extra full. When I pay attention to the feelings of satiety and stop eating at 5 or 6 on the hunger / satiety scale, I may feel more vulnerable. And at the same time I feel more open. That is usually nice; I feel alive but also a little tingly. But at times in life when I do not feel safe for some reason, it can be a bit uncomfortable.

I've found other ways to find that safety rather than stuffing myself in order to numb the tingle. To understand that the need for safety (or some other need) has been triggered, I have benefited greatly from using Tool 3 on page 45.

Week 3
Getting to know hunger

Take time to pause and consider about your hunger on at least five occasions this week. During these occasions, take 5-15 minutes to notice how it feels to be hungry. You don't have to be starving, but be somewhere between 2-4 on the hunger scale. It is probably a moment 2-4 hours since you last ate something. Maybe it is just before you are going to eat, or when you're about to prepare a meal.

Write down your observations and take a moment to reflect on what you have discovered.

Shorten the time between observing your hunger if the observation stimulates stronger emotions than what feels comfortable for you to manage on your own. Remember that this exercise is about getting to know your natural impulses better, not to change something, not to lose weight or get over something but about getting to know your own natural impulses better.

Regularly take your time to reflect on and answer these questions:

1. Where am I right now on the satiety/hunger scale? _____
2. Where in the body do I feel the hunger? Describe the feeling.
   Ask yourself:
- How do I know I'm hungry? Where in the body do I feel it? In the stomach? The neck? In my legs? Does it feel cold or hot? Is there any movement or stillness? Do I notice something else in my body?

3. What are my thoughts when I'm hungry? - Are they the same thoughts every time or do they differ from time to time?

4. Which of my needs are being met? (Use the list of need words on page 49).

5. Are there any of my needs that are not being met? What emotions are helping me to pay attention to those needs?

One challenge in using this scale is that many of us are not so familiar with the feeling of hunger that we can determine when we are truly hungry. Many of us confuse physical hunger with emotional hunger. We interpret other feelings as hunger or mix feelings of emotional hunger with those of physical hunger. Therefore, it is valuable to learn what characterizes hunger and satiety. Since the signs of fullness are delayed, it is valuable to learn to recognize the first signs that the body has gotten what it needs.

Take plenty of time for the first week's exercises and feel free to focus on them for a longer period if you need to.

There is a dilemma of sorts in suggesting that you eat between 2 and 5 on the scale, as all sorts of advice can easily become inner demands. Therefore notice all signs that you do not feel totally free and autonomous in your choices and remind yourself that you are always free to choose whatever you want.

What some people have said about the exercises from Weeks 1-3:

After doing the exercise on hunger a couple of times, I noticed that I often feel restless when I'm hungry. I also often get anxious and a little scared. I want to ACT. Perhaps it is natural, a struggle for survival?
Roger

When I tried to give myself time to feel my hunger, I realized that it's really scary to be hungry.
   Sonja

I'm more aware of how it is for me to be hungry after these exercises. I am grateful to gain awareness about this, so I can choose to eat when I'm hungry and not because it is "lunch time".
   Gertrud

An excerpt from a conversation between Susanne and me:
- It's hard for me to stop eating at five or six on the hunger / satiety scale. I stop at seven and usually begin on three.
- And you are not completely satisfied with that?
- I read that you suggested that it is best to eat between two and five on the scale. I'm worried that you're following my suggestion in a way that makes it a demand that you stop at five. I don't think it is particularly supportive to receive one more demand about how you should eat.
- Mm, it's easy to hear your suggestions as if I must stop at five or six.
- I wonder what it would take for you to accept for now that you can eat between three and seven?
-First of all, we can never know that we have the same experience of what a five or a six on the hunger scale really is. And the real aim of focusing on the hunger scale is to become aware of why you are eating. To become aware of the needs you are aiming to meet. Do you want to hear a few more thoughts I have around this?
- Yes.
- When you've reached what you call three and want to eat, to just pause and notice how hunger feels is a great first step. Then, if you eat more or not, it does not matter. This approach is a way to create balance, not to create control.
- Yes, that feels really good. How easy and obvious it suddenly became (laughter).

To eat when I'm hungry has not really settled in me yet. To plan the day around meals has always been deeply rooted in me. Often I think of the next meal before I've finished the one I'm in the middle of. To eat three times a day seems like a must, everybody does it, don't they. When I listened to my needs, I worried as I didn't seem to be hungry three times a day, but only two. I understand that the worry has more to do with conventions than about what my body actually needs, but still it bothers me.

Sara

Sara in the example above, discovered, as several others who have gone through the program in this book did, that she rarely let her hunger determine when she would eat. She had become accustomed to eat according to planned meal times, which meant she was not trained to be aware of hunger and fullness.

She rarely ate between meals, but she also was not observant to when she was satisfied as she ate her planned meals. It was as if an autopilot kicked in and it took a long time for her to really get to know her feelings of hunger and satiety. When she finally did, it was easy for her to feel more at ease finding her own meal times. She also lost the 10 kg, which she long had yearned to lose. This time without mortifying herself and without gaining weight as soon as the diet was over, as had happened so many times in the past.

Read more about how people experienced the exercises in the program on page 77.

Week 4
Follow Four Suggestions

Now that you've gotten to know your hunger and fullness levels, it is time to, over the next week, follow the four pieces of advice that are described in detail on page 11. If it feels too challenging to follow them throughout the week, go back to the exercises in weeks 1-3 or just choose a day when you:

1. Eat when you're hungry (whenever that happens during the day),
2. eat whatever you feel like,
3. enjoy what you chose to eat,
4. stop eating when you 're full.

If it feels challenging to quit, remind yourself of point 1 and that you can eat again whenever you are hungry. It might be supportive to keep a diary about what you learn from this, as this is a gradual process of learning to eat in a way that is more guided from within.

Use tools 1 and 2 on page 40 as an aid in any way you like and need help with.

If what you find most difficult for you is the first or the fourth pieces of advice, you might want to do the exercises in weeks 1-3 again to get to know hunger and fullness even deeper. If it, however, is the second or third pieces of advice that you find challenging, you can try the mindfulness exercise on page 62 before you proceed to the exercise in week 5.

Remember you do not have to be in a hurry with this process or program. This is not a slimming diet, not even a physical health one; it is an attempt to lay the foundations for a balanced and joyful way of eating that will last a lifetime.

Week 5

What needs am I trying to meet by eating?

The purpose of the exercise this week is to gain increased understanding of which needs you are trying to meet by eating. Start by using tool 3 on page 45. Take at least 15 minutes to fill it out and maybe change or add things in it during the week.

As often as it feels joyful and meaningful, ask yourself the question:
- *What are the needs I'm trying to meet by eating this? Make sure it is not hiding a demand to not eat something, but to really, as a first step, connect with the need.*

Ask yourself this when you shop, cook, when you put food on the plate, and when you put something in your mouth or after you have eaten.

Ask yourself after a meal, a snack or at the end of the day, if the needs you wanted to meet were met. Make it a game and absolutely do not interrogate yourself as if you were the food police.

Try to do it with warmth and curiosity. The aim is not to judge whether a choice of food or time to eat is right or wrong. The aim is to become more aware of your needs in relation to what you eat. In time, you can make the changes you want to make.

On some occasions you might want to restrain from eating something because you find that the need you want to meet is better met through some other strategy. During Week 6 you will be facing that challenge even more, so there is no reason to hurry.

Keep a diary of what and when you eat and which needs you are trying to satisfy by your eating. Do it one day or throughout the week.

You can also ask someone you trust, or often eat or hang out with, to ask the question about which needs you want to meet when you eat something. Make it clear to the person that the purpose is not to make you stop eating or refrain from something, but rather to become more conscious about needs. And that if they start making demands or expressing their opinion, it is the rebel in you that will be triggered and suddenly you will have eaten twice as much as you were intending to, in order to prove that you are free.

Week 6

Do my choices work?

Are there any needs that are not being met?

During this week, observe yourself in the same manner as during week 3: what needs you are trying to meet with eating. And this week, pay attention to if there are any needs that are not being met by what, how and when you eat. Use the list of needs on page 49 as support in your exploration.

Often the signals from needs that are not being met, are strongest at the end of a meal or shortly after you've eaten something. Sometimes they come as you lie down at night, when you relax and look back on your day. Perhaps the disappointment or frustration is greatest when you step on the scale or cannot get into your new pants. For some it may come as a sense of hopelessness and a sense of limitation.

You may notice that you feel depressed, restless or discontented. If you feel disappointment or disapproval of any kind after something you've eaten or not eaten, if possible take a moment to connect with what is going on within you. Remember that whatever feelings you might have, they can help you connect with your needs. Maybe you need to do some "detective work" and capture the thoughts buzzing in your head.

Behind all judgments are feelings and needs that are valuable to connect with. Take it gently. If you have tried disciplining and reprimanding yourself in order to gain control over what you have been eating over many years, this approach will shake your internal critic to the core.

The Critic may become noisy and raise all sorts of threats to make you regain control. Connect with what needs the critic want to remind you to also consider. Remember that you can go back to tool 2 on page 42. If you feel shame after eating, it is usually a sign that some needs were not met. Read more about shame on page 71.

Needbased Eating
Liv Larsson

Week 7

Do I want to choose something new?

Do I want to choose other strategies than eating to meet my needs?

Eating is a common strategy to meet needs other than obtaining nutrients or energy. Many people eat because it contributes to a sense of community and safety, but also because it provides a feeling of comfort and calm when one is emotionally upset.

Remember that there's nothing wrong with eating for these reason. But if some needs suffer because of how you choose to eat, you may want to makes some changes in your eating to include those needs as well. If you are not satisfied with how, when and what you eat in general, or on some certain occasion, try sometimes to do something else than eating at these times, and evaluate it afterwards if it was more satisfying. Saying I will not eat this is usually harder than saying, in order to meet this need I will do this or that.

Instead of saying "I will not eat now," determine what you actually want to do. Make a list of different things you could do to meet your needs. Enjoy the idea that there are actually many available options and that eating is only one of them. Experiencing freedom of choice makes it easier to see what you want.

Remember, I am not saying that you should refrain from eating something because you find that you eat for reasons other than for nourishment and energy. I want to help you become aware of your possible choices and that if you want, you can choose to eat something or not.

Beware of setbacks if you want to change something, because you think you have done something wrong or out of a "should". When we change something without embracing our need for autonomy we often rebel against it and can eat twice as much the next day.

Use tools 1-3 (page 38 - page 45) as support to make the changes you want to make.

Week 8

Be present with what it means to eat

During this week the goal is to increase your awareness of what is happening inside you before, during and after a meal. You can choose a particular day or a certain meal each day (for example, every lunch) when you focus particularly on this.

You can also choose to pay attention to your relationship with your eating during a certain time period during the day, for example between one and four o'clock each afternoon. Preferable, keep a diary so that you can more easily discover if there are any patterns around your way of eating.

This exercise, like the others in the program, is to simplify your life, not complicate it. If the exercise does not fit into your rhythm of life on this week, do it next week. Maybe you would rather put your time into doing the mindfulness exercise on page 35, to create more awareness around your eating.

I suggest that you read the questions below a few times during the week, so that you can find clarity about what you want to focus on. This is not about answering all the questions, but about focusing on your body and your mind to gain greater insight into how eating and food affects you. If it feels overwhelming to focus on several things at once, choose one or a couple of the questions and replace them with new ones when you feel you have found clarity around them.

- Pay attention to what you feel at the first thought of eating something. Is it hunger? Uneasiness? Restlessness? Boredom?
- When you are clear about what you feel, ask yourself what that feeling can tell you about what you need? Is it energy? Meaning? Community? Inspiration? Some other need?
- Is eating the most effective and meaningful way to address this need?
- What do you feel when you are about to eat this (if you decided to eat)? Is it joy? Eagerness? Hunger? Fatigue? Dissatisfaction?
- Do you take time to enjoy the flavors?
  - Is eating the way you want to meet those needs? Are there

other strategies that can also satisfy those needs, which may not be met by eating right now.- Are there strategies that also satisfy other needs, which may not be met by eating right now.

- What do you feel when you take the first bite?

- What do you feel while you eat?

- Are there any thoughts and feelings that recur while you are eating?

- How do you recognize that you are full?

- What are the first signs of being full? Where in the body do you feel that you are full? What do you do when you feel full?

Be gentle with yourself. Paying attention to what you feel does not mean that you are judging or criticizing the feelings or reactions. Just listen to your inner dialogue and to what you feel - the same way you would pay attention to a new acquaintance or a child you want to get to know. If the exploration creates stress or arouses strong emotions, you might want to go back to some exercise from the previous weeks. You might also share your feelings with someone that you think can be supportive.

If this exercise was especially valuable to you, you might want to do the mindfulness exercise on page 35 for a week before moving on to next week's exercise.

Week 9
Explore the Freedom of Choice

This week we will be focusing on something that concerns life-long learning - learning to listen to and to understand one's own inner critic. Our inner critic may have grown enormously if we have tried to follow a diet and failed. And if this has happened many times, it may be very loud. The smallest "mistake" or step outside of the diet can result in a lot of inner complaints. The critic's voice will always find something to criticize us for. Now it is time to try to understand what it really wants us to pay attention to.

Take the time this week to observe and write in your diary about your internal dialogue around food and weight. Listen especially to what your inner critic says about what you should eat, what you should refrain from eating, what you're not allowed to eat and what you'll have to stop eating all together. Write in your diary about the demands and "shoulds" that affect your sense of freedom.

Write down your critic's opinions about food, weight, body and other things that are challenging to hear. It is good for us to get to know our inner critics, as long as we keep in mind that what we want is to hear what it is trying to remind us of. The biggest problem is that the reminders usually come in a form that both tend to be painful and difficult to understand.

Perhaps you, like many others who have tried to control food and weight, have been tossed between control and failure, and back to control again. Our rancorous self-criticism may instead lead us to give up all attempts to control what we eat and we are left in rebellion against whatever "shoulds" we hear.

As the critic wants us to pay attention to our most important needs, make sure not to silence your critical voice, but to listen and try to understand the message behind it's voice. Pay attention to whether there are any new internal demands as a result of this program - the inner critic can turn anything against you - for example, telling you that you HAVE TO stop eating when you're full (because you interpret my proposal as demands).

Note after one week if there are any recurring demands or "musts". Ask yourself what needs these demands or accompanying criticism are trying to remind you about. Use the list of needs on page 49 as support. If you, for example, tell yourself that you should stop eating earlier, is it because it is a way for you to experience that your needs for hope or trust are met?

If, instead, your critic tells you that you SHOULD refrain from a sweet and fat dessert, is it perhaps to remind you that your health is important?

Once you have found which needs your inner critic wants to remind you of, try to find at least three different ways to meet those needs. One of the important things in creating balance in one's way of eating is to remember that there are always choices. Then the demands wither.

Week 10

Deepen your clarity around hunger and fullness

Choose one or more days this week when you will decide to eat as soon as you feel hunger that you would determine as 2 or 3 on the hunger/satiety scale on page 40.

Enjoy what you eat and pay attention to when you are at point 5 or 6 on the scale and then make a choice to stop eating there. Notice how it makes you feel. If you feel pressure around this, drop the exercise or return to it later in the week. This is an exploration and is not about achievement.

You can do the exercise below instead, or repeat the exercise for Week 9, to see if that gives you clarity about what is going on within you.

Maybe you want to read the short text about Change on page 29. Continue with this exercise for as many weeks that it feels meaningful. Do the exercise below at least once to get additional clarity.

When I did this exploration the first time I felt nothing special but I noticed after a few weeks that it had affected my attitude to hunger because I could more easily pay attention to the body's signals. One of the main insights was how hunger and satiety are so connected and are actually just different ends on the same scale. It also became clear to me that when I wait to eat until I am very hungry, it is much more likely that I will eat until I'm very full.

An exercise to make friends with feeling hungry or full:

1. Recall a recent time when you were very hungry. Sometime when you were on 1 or 2 on the hunger scale on page 40. Try to remember how and where in the body it felt and how it affected you emotionally. Take your time and let the memory be as clear as possible.

2. When this is clear, remind yourself of an occasion when you were stuffed. Maybe you would say that you were as high as an 8 or 9 on the scale. Try to remember how and where it felt in the body and how it affected you emotionally. Let the memory become clear in the same manner as in the first memory.

3. Ask yourself what was different about how these two situations felt. Then switch back and forth, preferably at least ten times between the two memories, and compare them with each other until they are very clear to you. Take plenty of time and notice both large and small differences. Try not to judge but to just explore.

Week 11

Find a Natural Way of Eating

During yet another week use the four suggestions below. If it is challenging to follow them throughout the week go back to any previous exercise, or choose a day when you follow the advice to:

1. Eat when you are hungry.
2. Eat whatever you feel like.
3. Enjoy what you eat.
4. Stop eating when you're full.

If this seems too challenging or stressfull, remind yourself of point 1 and that whenever you are hungry you will eat again. Write in your diary about what you learn from this to get an overview. Also take some time to read more about the above four suggestions as they are desribed earlier in the book.

Use tools 1 and 2 on page 40 as support. Remember that you do not need to hurry. It is not a health or slimming diet. The intention is to lay the foundations for balanced eating that hopefully will last a lifetime.

Week 12

Deepened Hunger and Satiety

Use the hunger / satiety scale again. Recognize as often as possible during the week where you are on the scale. Put the image of the scale somewhere where you can see it often. At any time during the day when you remember it, look at the scale and note the number you would say describes your level of hunger/satiety at that moment.

I suggest that you keep some kind of diary around hunger/satiety to see if there are any patterns around, for example, the times when you notice hunger. What thoughts around food usually turn up at a certain time? What feelings other than hunger? If you want, you can consciously use at least one day this week when you try to eat as soon as you are somewhere between point 2-3.

Make it a point to enjoy what you eat and pay attention to when you are at point 5 or 6 and then stop eating. Notice how it makes you feel.

After this week evaluate how you want to continue your exploration. Maybe you feel that you've built up the internal support you need and can let go of studying this. Maybe you want to deepen your insights and do part of the program again.

One way to evaluate where you are at now is to fill in tool 3 and compare it with the answers from earlier times when you filled it in. If you haven't done the mindfulness exercise on page 40, you may want to try that. Whatever you do, I hope you'll find many ways to meet your life-giving needs.

Evaluation

After doing the exploration in the program it is useful to return to tool 3. Note if anything has changed since you used it the first time. The questions below are a bit simplified, use them or the ones in Tool 3.

1. What needs are you trying to meet by eating?
2. Choose one of these needs.
3. Think of a time when that need was met.
4. What do you feel when you connect with this need?
5. What else can you do than eat to meet this need?
6. How do you feel when you think of these strategies? Is there a sense of freedom of choice? Is there a sense of should or of a demand to act in a certain way?

Use questions 2-6 with as many needs as you feel like. If you still don't experience the change that you are looking for, read the part about change on page 29.

Eating and shame

Shame is a topic that everyone who wants to make some changes in their eating may benefit from understanding more about. Many of us are driven by shame. We are ashamed of how we eat and how we look and we try to do a lot of things to avoid the grueling feeling of shame. One sign that we eat out of emotional hunger is that we feel shame or guilt after eating.

A man I once regularly coached had long suffered from the extra kilos he carried around. He also suffered from not living the way he wanted to live. Often he criticized himself and said that he did not contribute sufficiently to others and to the world at large. He often withdrew and wrestled with his inner critic.

When during one of our conversations he realized how much shame ruled his life, and that there were important needs behind the shame, everything shifted. He discovered how he longed for integrity and to be proud of the way he lived his life. We did not talk with each other for several months after that due to different reasons. One day I heard from him and he told me what the contact with the need for integrity had led to. He had begun to make more conscious choices in different areas of his life.

In at least 9 times out of 10 when he normally would have bought something to eat in a way he later would experience a lack of integrity around, he now did something different. He noted the cost of what he wanted to buy and then took that money and sent it to a project he wanted to support. Both of these choices contributed strongly to self-reliance and helped him to live and act with integrity.

Shame is so central in our lives that many of us have not even discovered how our eating is affected by it. Therefore, it is usually worthwhile to take a moment to think about how shame and your desire to eat in a more free and balanced manner are intertwined. I would like to ask you to read a piece of advice. My hope is that you see it as an interesting challenge to explore. If you notice that you see it as self-criticism, please let it go.

Do not eat to avoid shame, but do not refrain from eating for the same reason. In short: Do not eat to avoid feeling shame or to push shame away. Also do not refrain from eating to avoid shame.

One thing I discovered when I was working with my own approach to eating and my body, but also when I have been supporting others, is that we usually want to handle it on our own. People have often been walking around for years with anxiety about their weight or their way of relating to food before seeking support from others.

Shame is often involved in our approach to our body, our weight and to food. To ask what someone weighs can be more charged than to ask what their monthly salary is or how old they are - which are loaded subjects for many people.

Shame can be a part of "the recovery" if we dare to embrace it. And I mean - really embrace and feel it. In my book, Anger, Guilt and Shame, Reclaiming Power and Choice, I have described in detail how we can befriend our shame[7].

To get there, we first need to realize what we are doing to avoid shame. We can summarize the most common choices into four categories. I have summarized them under the name "compass of needs," because with the help of the four different directions of the compass we can understand our underlying needs.

1. **We withdraw.**
2. **We minimize and criticize ourselves.**
3. **We rebel against the shame and do what we fear or that someone says is not ok.**
4. **We criticize or minimize others.**

1. To withdraw:

There are many who shy away from parties, bathing and exercise

---

7 Larsson, Liv (2010) Anger, guilt and shame, Reclaiming Power and Choice.

in order to avoid feeling shame about their bodies. We refrain from things that could bring joy, togetherness and enjoyment because of this. Feelings of shame can convert a beach to a hell rather than a place to go to on vacation for people who are obese - imagined or real – as they are often reluctant to show their bodies.

It is not only obesity that may prevent it, but also that we think that we're not perfect in some way or another. Even people who are thin or have other complexes about their bodies can withdraw to avoid having to feel shame.

Another way to withdraw has to do with clothing. We might dress in a way that makes us almost invisible, or we might do everything possible to hide our body, although we would much rather dress differently. We do not want to take any risk of feeling more shame. Another way to withdraw is to refrain from intimacy and sex.

During a period when I felt really badly and had the most anxiety about my weight and body,

I had a distorted image of my body. I experienced myself as fat even though I was very thin.

I sometimes chose to withdraw physically, but more often, I was present physically but not psychologically. Binge eating is often done in solitude as a real act of withdrawal.

When I ate stealthily, there was a thought that I was also able to sneak away from how the food would affect my weight or my health. If no one saw it, it had never happened. This made it almost an adventure, something exciting, something that, at least temporarily, led to an experience of freedom and autonomy. I was the one in control of my life! I felt such a sweet sense of power.

I became giggly, excited and very attentive when I ate stealthily, attentive on anything else than what I ate that is. But unfortunately, the resulting costs are usually considerably higher than the excitement of the moment. Guilt and shame, coupled with disappointment and resignation is often the cost. So start at once by asking yourself - what needs do you want to meet by eating when no one else is watching?

When you gulp down a chocolate bar in the car or eat something sweet midway between two meetings, check in on yourself about how you feel? Or maybe you want to take it even further and "Sneak knowingly" to gain clarity about what is going on inside. Buy something, candy for example, that you hide away as soon as you've paid for it. Then eat what you bought on the sly, maybe inside the washroom or behind some other locked door.

Eat quickly and silently. Choose a "forbidden" item to eat and the most forbidden place to eat it in. Do it consciously and try to really enjoy the experience. Ask yourself how it makes you feel? What important needs do you want to meet so much that you hide away from others when you eat? Are there needs that are greatly unmet in your life at the moment? Is there any way to satisfy them with another strategy than to eat stealthily?

Remember to use these questions as a way to get to know yourself better, and not from a thought that eating in this way would be wrong. If you have a thought that it is wrong to withdraw and eat, embrace that thought and ask what need you are worried will not be met by it.

2. To minimize criticize and attack ourselves:

One way to try to avoid shame is by minimizing ourselves and continually commenting on how ugly or fat we are. The self-criticism makes the feeling of shame more bearable and we do not need to withdraw. We can participate at parties or go to the beach if we just keep it clear to ourselves that we are not okay.

Through self-criticism, we defend ourselves from attacks from others by ridiculing or blaming ourselves first. But at least we are taking part in the community.

To binge eat or starve oneself is a form of violence against ourselves. It begins as an attempt to meet our needs but it takes on a destructive expression. It provides, however, a temporary break from the shame.

In my teens, my inner critic was often busy criticizing my body, my way of eating or my weight. "Ugly and fat" echoed in my head, "ugly and fat, ugly and fat, ugly and fat." During periods when I was in touch with what I needed and acted to meet all my needs, it was able to take a vacation, as it was no longer needed to keep me alert. But as soon as I was not willing to embrace shame and transform it to other feelings and to needs, the inner critic started working again. In this way shame had become a friend who reminded me to take care of some needs that I had forgotten.

Many of us are at war with our bodies. To avoid shame we might call our body's names we would never accept others to use about us. We might criticize the way we look in ways that we would never dream of doing to someone else. We will eat food or candy we would not like to feed our children out of concern for their health. In many cases, it is a way of dealing with shame, but at the cost of both health and self-trust.

3. To rebel against shame and do what we fear the most

Some of us do the opposite of withdrawing when we feel shame and vulnerability. We step forward, invading any feeling of shame as if we want to show the world around us that we are invincible. We no longer feel the shame but rebel against every prohibition. Maybe we dress in a challenging way or in a manner that signals that we do not care at all about appearance.

I was binge eating and starving myself in my teenage years for quite a long time without anyone knowing about it. This alternated with periods when I rebelled and did things to show that "I'm not afraid of anything." I hitchhiked alone through the Sahara desert and wandered and rode without a Chinese visa in Tibet in the mid eighties and a lot of other things where I exposed myself to great danger. I invaded my shame, pushed away the space where self-care could have been and became hard, cold and most of all disconnected.

For long periods during those years, I avoided shame, invading any trace of weakness, so much so that I did not need to binge-eat, as I was too busy rebelling against all prohibitions. However, it was very lonely and not sustainable in the long run.

4. Minimizing or attacking others

When we are not able to bear the shame within ourselves anymore, and cannot cope with the constant blaming of ourselves, we can choose to attack others. We might make nasty comments about people we see as fat or people we think are working out excessively. We might indulge in opinions such as "fat people are nice and thin people are mean" or vice versa depending on the category in which we place ourselves.

We might claim that fat people are smart or stupid, depending on what suits us. The core of it all, however, is to try to escape from the shame we feel inwardly by attacking outwardly. Just as in the other three categories of the compass of needs, this strategy will only work for a while to keep the shame away. Unfortunately we can have created conflicts and distanced ourselves from people who otherwise could have been important to us through our behavior and aggression.

Afterword

This book is based on the idea that our body knows how to regulate its food intake in relation to the energy we burn. But with all that we have learned about what is right and wrong to eat, many of us have lost some of this natural approach.

My hope is that through this book you have gotten back some trust in this natural ability. I feel happy to have had the chance to share some tools that have changed so much for me. What earlier was something that often stole the joy of life has become an exciting – if yet sometimes challenging - area to focus on. I hope with all my heart that you have found more freedom, balance and enjoyment by using this book.

Voices from people who have used the exercises:

"When I realized how often I ate to relax, I began to regularly take a 10 minute break as often as I could. I also took a moment of silence just before a meal. This reduced stress around food and I could make a more aware choice of what I chose to eat."

"When I understood that I had something sweet with my coffee because I was sad or worried and that I often was even more down afterwards, I decided instead to call a friend who I know can listen. The craving always went away when I managed to talk to someone."

"It was frustrating to realize how often I eat because I do not want to feel restless. Eating was set on autopilot. I numbed all sorts of emotions with food and sweets. When I realized that in those situations, I usually had a need of more meaning and for inspiration, it was clear that I would get more out of reading a book or talking to someone I have inspiring conversations with."

"I'm ashamed to tell you that I noticed that I often ate candy or some snack like potato chips when I had a need to be seen and heard. Often it happened after I had been standing in front of a group and felt a little lonely and outside the group. The goodies did not help, but numbed the longing for closeness a bit. Now I see that I actually have many other options that meet my needs even better."

"When I realized my need for community was a major motivational force in taking a coffee break, I decided to be more active in inviting others along when I went to a café. This meant that cakes and sweets were no longer important and sometimes were replaced by a walk with a friend."

"When I saw that my need for freedom of choice and to know that I can live my own dreams were behind my decisions to eat things I had decided were "banned," I could more often pause, get in touch with the fact that it was I who chose what to eat and to make more aware choices. Sometimes I eat what I previously called 'forbidden fruit' and I enjoy it so much more. Sometimes I refrain from eating it and realize that I am more at ease at all levels by eating something else."

"I have discovered that it is not food or weight that is my problem. It's that I do not value and prioritize socializing and things I find fun."

Litterature and references

Berg, Lasse (2011) Dawn Over the Kalahari.

Diamond, Jared (1999), Guns, Germs and Steel. WW Norton & Co.

Haskvitz, Sylvia (2005), Eat By Choice, Not By Habit. Puddle Dancer Press.

McKenna, Paul (2005) I Can Make You Thin, Bantam Press.

Orbach, Susie (2014) Fat is a Feminist Issue. Arrow Books Ltd.

Larsson, Liv (2011), Anger, Guilt and Shame, Reclaiming Power and Choice. Friare Liv.

Liedloff, Jean (1986), The Continuum Concept: In Search of Happiness Lost(Classics in Human Development) Da Capo

Lyubomirsky, Sonja (2009), The How of Happiness: A New Approach to Getting the Life You Want. Penguin.

Rosenberg, Marshall (2004), Getting Past the Pain Between Us: Healing and Reconciliation without Compromise.

Rosenberg, Marshall (2007), Nonviolent Communication,
A Language for Life. Puddle Dancer Press.

Stopping Emotional Eating. Heartmath.org

Stahre och Ryd (2012) Snällfällan: att bryta med känslomässigt ätande. Bonnier fakta.

Thich Nhat Hanh & Cheung. (2011) Savor: Mindful Eating, Mindful Life. HarperOne.

For mer information about NVC
www.friareliv.se
www.nonviolentcommunication.se
www.cnvc.org

About the author

Liv Larsson

For over 10 years Liv suffered from eating disorders. She has tried most diets, exercised and been crazily committed to "becoming thin". She has also violently opposed it all, rebelled against all diets and remedies, and finally decided to write a book about what she has discovered.

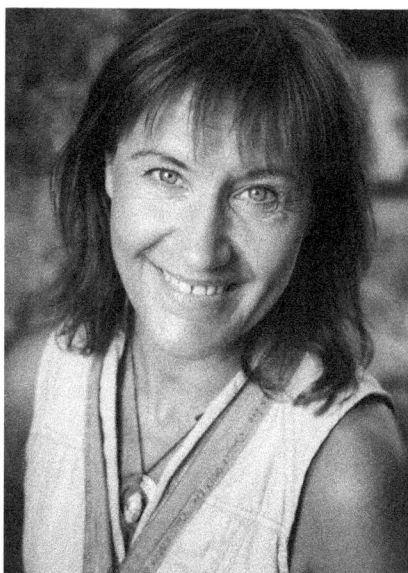

For more than 30 years, Liv has led groups, teaching communication, conflict management and mediation. Since 1999 she has worked with Nonviolent Communication and is a certified trainer with CNVC. She educates and works as a mediator in Sweden as well as internationally. Liv has written 15 books including 3 for children, many of them translated into different languages.

Find more info about Liv:
www.friareliv.se/eng
www.livlarsson.com
www.cnvc.org

Other titles in english by Liv Larsson

Cracking the Communication Code. 42 Key Differentiations in NVC.
Co-authored with Katarina Hoffmann. 2014

The Power of Gratitude. 2014.

Anger, Guilt and Shame, Reclaiming Power and Choice. 2013.

A Helping Hand. Mediation with Nonviolent Communication. 2011.

Relationships – Freedom without Distance, Belonging without Control. 2012.

Read more and get your copy at www.friareliv.se/books

www.ingramcontent.com/pod-product-compliance
Lightning Source LLC
Chambersburg PA
CBHW030028290326
41934CB00005B/537